VEGAN DIET FOR BEGINNERS

Adopting A Vegan Diet For Weight Loss & Good Mental Health!

By

KATYA JOHANSSON

Table Of Contents

Introduction

How and why veganism started was filled with fascinating source material that covers expert about the diet. Dr. John McDougall is an advocate of consuming a diet, full of starch, to fight devastating diseases such as cancers, sclerosis and diabetes.

A vegan diet means that you eat no animal products containing dairy products. Eradicating what makes up the majority of foods used up in the typical American diet can be extremely overwhelming. My first suggestion is transition in steps and don't do it all at once. Take a slow start.

Even if you're not involved in the vegan diet this book is a great addition to your collection due to the informative section about desires. Ever have those desires for something crispy, or sweet and salty for some chocolate? Well, these needs are described in detail and suggests a healthy alternative that recognizes the vitamin deficiency and the food that would address that desire.

For instance, have an impulsive desire for chocolate? It means our body might actually be craving magnesium which can be found in seeds, nuts, fruit and Legumes. Are you craving for sweet or sugary foods? Then your body might require carbon, sulfur, phosphorus or chromium. These vitamins are found in fresh fruits and broccoli just to name a few.

Why I Wrote This Book

With passage of time, I've been considering a lot about this space and what I can do in the New Year to challenge myself in new techniques. I often struggle with questions like – What can I do to make a difference? What should I do to help people and animals? Am I growing on just for myself?

Unluckily, these questions have gone mostly unanswered. Don't get me wrong, I love to
share my recipes with you, so I have no plans to quit recipe development. It's something I enjoy a lot. But there are few things I could be doing and I've felt this in my heart a lot in recent months. I'm feeling tired and I'm sure this a big reason for the rut I'm stuck in. The good thing is that it usually prompts a change for the better.

In essence of change, I'm initiating a series on veganism this year that can make the transition to a vegan diet easier. I'm really enthusiastic about this. To be honest, it's something I've craved to do for over a year now, but I have the mindset that if I can't do it accurately or if I don't know all the answers, then I shouldn't do it. Well, this is a pretty silly way to go through life, don't you think? The truth is, I'm the only one holding myself. I want to share whatever it is that I can offer and faith that it will be useful for some of you. Even if you have no craving of going vegan or if you are already a vegan, I still expect that this series will be inspirational and peak some inquisitiveness about things you may want to know more about.

It happened to me that it would be more useful if I write my experiences in the book. If there's one thing I've known over the past few years, it's that a vegan food isn't about what you take away; it's really about what you add in. I didn't aware of this for a long time.

For every food that I decided to relinquish, I added at least a few of new, energetic foods in its place. But first, I had to know what it is I could add into my diet. This wasn't easy for me in the start and I was uncertain it's not for many. Three years into it, I'm still very much learning.

To make this book a success, it's important for me to have your feedback. I'd love to know some of the questions you are wanting right now or perhaps things you struggled with in the past.

Everyone loves a good success story, including me.

Why should you Read this Book

This book is the vital book for learning about the benefits of a vegan diet. It will helped you understand the science behind a vegan diet and showed to you that veganism was the way to go.

The books explains in simple terms how a vegan diet is the sturdiest tool we have against disease and ailment. It is easy to read and will entirely change how you ponder about food. You'll be hooked by the Introduction where the book tells you that by simply changing your diet, you can completely avoid heart disease, diabetes, and obesity.

He also reexamines the myth about protein and depicts how not only vegans are getting sufficient protein, but that eating a lot of protein actually promotes cancer. This book teaches you how to eat in order to make your health best and longevity, and tells why you haven't been educated proper diet before. The book lastly looks at the frightening truth as to why there is so much distortion about how we should be eating.

This is a fantastic cookbook for a beginner in the vegan cooking world. Not only are the recipes delicious and tasty, but the directions are easy to read and the ingredients are easy to get. Most of the recipes take very short time to make, making this cookbook vital for the busy vegan.

Chapter 1: What is Veganism?

The vegan diet was defined early in 1944, it was as late as 1949 before Leslie J Cross exposed that a definition of veganism was needed by the society. He suggested the principle of the freedom of animals from exploitation by man.

This is later made clear as to seek an end to the use of animals by man for diet, goods, work, hunting, and by all other uses involving misuse of animal life by man.

Veganism is a way of living which seeks to exclude, as far as is possible and feasible, all kinds of exploitation of, and brutality to, animals for food, clothing or all other purpose.
There may be some distinctions sometimes made between several categories of veganism.

Dietary vegans also called as strict vegetarians stop eating animal products, not only meat but also eggs, dairy products, and other animal-derived substances. And dietary vegans are often focused on the health features of whole foods, and, as such, may take in honey or clothing that contain animal products (for instance, leather or wool).

The term ethical vegan is more applied to those who do not only follow a vegan diet and oppose the use of animal products for any purpose. Another term, often used, is environmental veganism, which states the prevention of use of animal products.

Chapter 2: Reasons to Go Vegan Today

Veganism used to be the monarchy of hippies and Hindus but today, it's dominating the world. From California to Calcutta, people are quitting meat for health, environmental, economic and ethical causes and the fact is that veganism is a great approach to the diet resolutions.

In fact, there are loads of great causes to quit meat, dairy and eggs. But veganism isn't just about your food – why not quitting wearing fur and leather, too?

The good news is that it is easy to go vegan. In the 1970's, only approx. 1% of Americans were vegetarian. By 2013, 13% of Americans were vegetarian and 7% were vegan. This shows you can find vegan options in supermarkets and restaurants, and even some vegan fast food. Now so many people going vegan.

If you're still not inspired, we've come up with 12 solid reasons to go vegan. You only need one good cause to change your lifestyle, and there's no better time to start improving your health. If you're already vegan, why not share this book with someone who's not? Perhaps, it is just the nudge they need

1. Long Life

Plenty of studies have proved that vegans are less likely to contract the main lethal diseases in the West: heart disease, cancer, diabetes, and high blood pressure. Despite what people believe, vegans can get all the nourishments that they require to be healthy from their food, including protein, fiber, and minerals, without all the bad stuff that meat has, like hormones, antibiotics and the bad kinds of saturated fat.

2. Slimmer and Smarter

The famous singer Beyoncé said even after going on some crazy dieting routine, she still couldn't lose weight until she went vegan. Vegans are, on average, up to 10 kg lighter than carnivores are.

Some people believe going vegan is only about rice, pasta, bread ,nut loafs and vegan cheesecakes. Be sure to observe the carbs and calories, and also make sure you're getting lots of vegan proteins like tofu, hemp protein powder and quinoa.

3. Healthy Planet

Eating meat and wearing leather are not healthy activities. These activities are actually inefficient and cause massive amounts of pollution and the meat industry is also one of the biggest reasons of climate change. Taking a vegan diet is more even more effective than all kinds of other foods.

4. Save Animals

This seems obvious, but do you know that each vegan protects the lives of more than hundred animals a year? Some may argue that if the animals are treated with kindness and gentleness, then it is ok.' This is simply not the case with meat, and organic dairy and eggs are still produced in a painful manner. There is no easier way to help animals and avoid suffering than by choosing vegan foods as alternative to meat, eggs, and dairy products.

5. Yummy and Easy

Veganism is certainly mainstream now, and dairy-product alternatives are very common. Pizzerias now offer vegan cheese pizzas, and there are tofu containing burgers that taste like the real thing.

6. Meat, sometimes disgusting

Meat is sometimes contaminated with feces, blood, and other harmful fluids as animal products account for the biggest source of food poisoning in the USA. And by meat, we're not just considering beef here. Some scientists at the Johns Hopkins Bloomberg School of Public Health verified supermarket chickens and found that 96 percent of Tyson chicken was replete with campylobacter, a dangerous bacteria that causes 2.4 million cases of food poisoning every year, causing diarrhea, cramping, abdominal pain, and fever.

7. Dairy as Source of Pus and Blood

According to Élise Desaulniers, there are ten myths about the dairy industry, milk and cheese are replete with hormones, antibiotics and some organic dairy may have pus and blood. Many people are allergic to lactose and will confront gas, bloating and tummy aches after eating dairy products. Milk products also boost the production of mucous in our bodies, which is kind of gross. Despite what cheese lovers may tell you, dairy is not the best way to get calcium in your food; almost all leafy greens, almonds, broccoli and many soya products as soy yogurt are a important way to get this mineral.

8. Vegan fashion

Ms. McCartney verified that vegan fashion may be very stylish, loads of designers have trailed. Some important brands are matching and exceeding the looks of mainstream designers who insist on fashion.

9. How Flesh is formed

According to Peta and Cowspiracy, consuming meat doesn't just hurt animals but it also hurts people. It needs tons of crops and water to raise animals. In reality, it takes up to 6 kg of grain to yield just 1 pound of animal flesh. All that vegan food could be used efficiently if it were fed straight to people. The more people go to vegan, the better able we'll be to feed the world.

10. Save Money

Meat and cheese are the most expensive things in the in our lives. By going to vegan proteins, you will save a lot.

11. You're in good company

People are making the switch to a vegan lifestyle including some of the planet's famous stars.

Joaquin Phoenix, Natalie Portman, Ariana Grande, Liam Hemsworth and Ellie Goulding are a few stars who have decided not to make their bodies a graveyard for dead animals.

12. it's not a religion

If you go out with friends at night and they order a pizza, and that mozzarella looks very tasty right now...eat it. Going vegan does not mean that if you have leather boots or eat a piece of cake that was made with eggs you will go straight to vegan hell. The basic idea is to try to do the best you can, and to keep in mind that every little change helps not only you and the animals, but the every creature on the planet as a whole too.

13. Glowing skin

Forget expensive potions and lotions with the idea that ditching dairy can give you the best skin of your life.

Various studies have found that dairy ingestion can cause and increase the severity of acne.

This could be down to a number of aspects, from dairy products producing skin inflammation to the fact that milk has some hormones which may affect the skin.

Chapter 3: The Do's and Don'ts of a Vegan Lifestyle

Vegetarian diets come in many forms. The types vary from super strict to really flexible and everything in between. If you're attracted towards the lingo: Vegans eat no animal products at all, while others like ovo-lacto vegetarians take in eggs and dairy. Pescatarians are ovo-lacto vegetarians that also consume fish, and flexitarians consume mainly vegetarian meals, but rarely include other non-vegetarian foods, such as a grass fed beef sometimes.

As dietitians, our jobs are to assist people find the diet that suits their preferences and way of life best it should be well-balanced, tastes superb, and is fulfilling their nutrient needs. Often this means working to put together balanced vegetarian diets. So whatever your preference of vegetarianism, here are the vital Dos and Don'ts you'll want to study if you're following a vegetarian lifestyle.

Don't...

Rely on packaged vegan foods.

Many pre-packaged vegan foods are replete with with artificial elements and sodium, and most are high in calories. If you examine the packaging, you may be astonished to know that many veggie burgers are higher in calories than a beef patty and may also have extra chemicals to make it tasty and colorful. Take in packaged vegan foods no more than once a week.

Forget about the protein.

Animal-based foods are higher in protein, so you should replace them with high-protein vegan alternatives. Veggies like beans, soymilk, quinoa, tofu, peanut butter and oatmeal are all good sources of protein. Examine these surprising sources of protein for some more ideas (but note that not all of them are vegan-friendly).

Just eat raw food.

Some vegans like eating raw foods. In most cases, cooked vegetables, beans and grains are easier for our bodies to digest and can give us more nutrients. Mix raw and cooked food for a healthy balance.

Do eat whole plant-based foods

The advantage of going vegan come from not only eradicating animal-based ingredients, but also from eating a wide variety of unprocessed nutrient-rich plant-based foods, containing fruits, veggies, whole grains like quinoa, lentils, nuts, beans, seeds, herbs, spices, and healthy plant fats, such as coconut and avocado. Similarly a white bagel with margarine is vegan, but it's not nourishing or good for you. Make quality vegan foods your focus.

DON'T load up on vegan junk food

There are lot of vegan products in the market, it's easy to be a junk food vegan. Some years ago vegans made most of their meals from scratch. Nowadays, there's a large supply of highly processed vegan foods, from delicious pepperoni pizza and fake bacon to healthy vegan cookies, candy, and donuts. I've seen many vegans who never eat fruits and veggies, and some others who live off of sweet potato chips and licorice. Vegan treats such as ice cream made from coconut milk are good in balance, but the bulk of your meals and snacks should be include nutrient-packed whole foods.

DO drink plenty of water

Healthfully going vegan means you'll have your intake of both, in addition to some fiber-rich foods, like beans and nuts. This dietary change could easily result in doubling or tripling your daily fiber consumption and that means you'll need plenty of water. Your body won't be able to break down the fiber in food, and consume it from your digestive tract into your bloodstream, so the fiber should work its way through your system in order to be eradicated. Water always helps move it through, so at least 16 ounces, four times a day.

DON'T forget about protein

Protein gives building blocks that maintain and repair your tissues of body, comprising of muscle, hormones, and enzymes. It also boosts satiety, and revs up metabolism. Without protein in your food, you will feel fatigued, get sick often, and notice a drying of your skin and hair. Vegan foods can give enough, but it is important to have protein sources in every meal. Quinoa gives 8 grams per cup; almonds approx. 7.5 g per quarter cup whole; lentils 17 g per cup; and a vegan protein powder, like pea protein, can have about 25 grams per scoop.

Do Veganize Usual Meals

We should replace the meat and dairy with vegan diet. For instance, stuff peppers with lentils in place of ground turkey, and add cannellini beans to a soup instead of chicken, and make chili with kidney beans in place of beef. In almost any dish, from tacos to stir-fry's, you can switch meat, poultry or seafood with beans or lentils. To substitute dairy, choose milks made from almonds, coconut, or sunflower seeds, and use some more virgin olive or coconut oil in place of butter. Instead of creamy dressings like Caesar and ranch, try to use tahini.

DON'T forget about ethnic eateries

Some of people worry that going vegan make it difficult to dine out, but in many societies, vegan dishes are staples. Some of my favorites comprise of Indian (chana masala), Middle Eastern (hummus and tabbouleh), and Thai (green curry).

Chapter 4: Best Approach for weight loss on a vegan diet

I want to stress that the vegan diet can be unhealthy and can cause weight gain, especially if you are just consuming vegan processed food and spaghetti all day. But, compared to an omnivore food, a vegan diet is good for weight loss due to these reasons:

1. Lower in fat, cholesterol and calories

There are definitely some health advantages of eating organic, grass-fed meat, most people are consuming much meat. Meat contains saturated cholesterol, fat and a lot of calories. Depending on reasons like muscle mass and whether you are working out, the body only consumes about 20-30 grams of protein at a time, which means the rest of protein gets stored as fat. Consider now that a 100gram of chicken has about 25 grams of protein. That's large quantity of protein which is turning into fat.

By comparing, vegan sources of protein are low in fat, have very little saturated fat and cholesterol, and have often much lower calories. As vegan foods have high fiber, they make you feel satisfied for longer so you don't need as many calories to feel satisfied. And, it is easier to get sufficient protein on the vegan food.

2. No Hormones

One of the big problems with consuming meat and animal products is that steroid hormones are often utilized in production. The companies give the animals hormones like progesterone, estrogen, and their artificial versions to make cows grow faster and give more milk. Those hormones which are produced to make cattle gain weight swiftly and also affect humans too.

The World Health Organization, have accepted the connection between hormones in meat and fatness.

3. Vegan Diet Creates Food Awareness

The main reason why the vegan food is good for weight loss is because it creates food awareness. When you go vegan, one of the first changes you notice is that shopping takes a lot longer as you have to spend so much time in reading diet labels to check animal ingredients inside. It won't take long before you know that virtually all processed foods are mixed with junk like high fructose corn syrup and hydrogenated oil, all of which are cause of weight gain and obesity.

Food awareness helps people make better food choices.

4. Don't Count Calories but Eat Real Food

One of the important things about the vegan weight loss food is that you need not count calories. Studies show that counting calories can make you fat.

The reason that counting calories for weight loss doesn't work is because:

It sometimes makes diet seem like a chore
It is almost impossible to count calories accurately
A calorie is, in fact, not just a calorie

6. Don't Replace Meat

There is one rule of happy veganism. Don't think you're eating cow. No matter how much you work on tofu or wheat gluten, it will never taste like a Big Mac. So stick with a veggie-based protein and a grain, and know that's taking you towards your weight loss goals. You'll find new flavors that will slim you down.

7. Power up with plant based protein powder

You can't eat or drink whey or egg protein powder on a vegan food and that is why you're losing weight. Researchers exposed that people who consumed higher amounts of plant protein were far less liable to metabolic syndrome, in a 2015 study in the Journal of Diabetes Investigation. In another study in Nutrition Journal found that plant protein ingestions may play a role in stopping obesity.

Conclusion

A vegan diet has the ability to transform your life and rejuvenate your body. By eating the foods we were naturally designed to eat – the body can really function properly. You can be more alert, slim & happy. In addition, some people report a higher sex drive on a plant based diet as well.

If you consider veganism, start slow. Adapt some recipes you like and find their vegan version. Eat as much as your body needs, but make sure you stay away from oils and vegan junk food. Stick to natural whole foods.

To Your Successful Journey,
Katya Johnasson.